Longevity Guide

Journey to centenarians

By

Clark Tyler

Table of contents

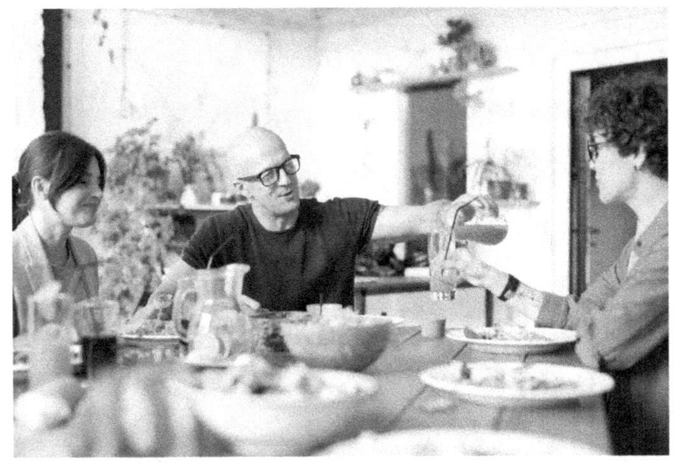

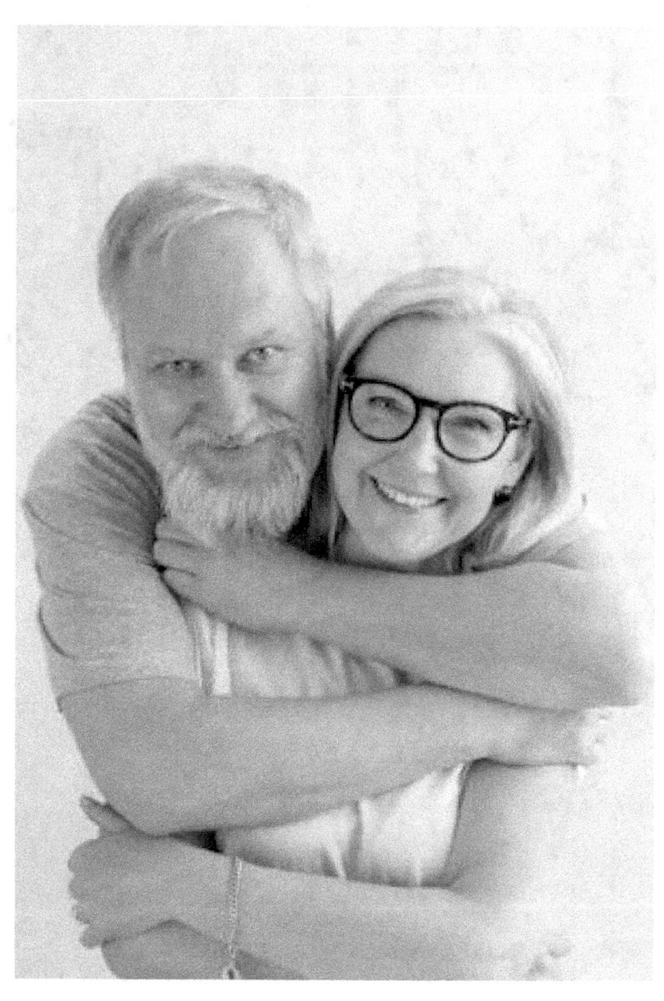

Introduction

Brief overview of the importance of longevity

The idea of longevity, or living a long and healthy life, is crucial for many facets of personal health and social advancement. Personal growth, desire fulfillment, and the pursuit of varied experiences are all made possible by living longer. It offers the chance to see and participate in the development of generations, promoting a feeling of continuity and interconnectedness. Longevity and medical science breakthroughs are closely related from a health standpoint. Alongside efforts to increase life expectancy, society is also focused on improving the quality of those extra years. This quest has produced ground-breaking results in customized healthcare, preventative medicine, and cutting-edge therapies for age-related illnesses. The desire to live a longer life has sparked an investigation into the complexities of aging with the goal of discovering the mechanisms behind metabolic resilience and cellular regeneration. From an economic perspective, longevity is a key factor in determining the demographic composition. Longer lifespans result in a workforce with greater experience and competence, which might increase productivity and spur economic growth. It does, however, present certain difficulties, such as the requirement for long-term healthcare systems and pension plans in order to maintain an aging population. Moreover, longevity has significant social consequences. It modifies established systems, making people reevaluate their retirement, employment, and educational options. Longevity calls into question assumptions about life phases and forces society to change by fostering circumstances that support lifelong learning and a variety of professional paths. In summary, longevity is a complex idea with wide-ranging effects, rather than just an individual goal. Its importance spans economic dynamics, societal growth, healthcare improvements, and personal contentment. In our dynamic environment, recognizing and appreciating longevity is crucial to promoting holistic approaches to both individual and societal well-being.

concept of maintaining and enhancing health

A fundamental idea that goes beyond personal well-being is that sustaining and improving health shapes social structures and impacts the course of human development. Fundamentally, health is a dynamic condition of physical, mental, and social well-being rather than just the absence of sickness. In order to achieve optimal health, one must adopt a proactive, holistic approach that recognizes the interdependence of all aspects of life. When it comes to personal wellbeing, being healthy is like building a strong base that enables people to overcome obstacles in life. Vitality and energy are derived from physical health, which is defined as sufficient rest, a balanced diet, and frequent exercise. Concurrently, a happy and meaningful existence depends on mental health, which includes both emotional stability and cognitive ability. Understanding the mutually beneficial link between mental and physical health emphasizes the value of complete self-care techniques. The idea of health has an impact on social structures and economic processes in addition to the person. Populations in good health are more productive, which promotes stability and growth in the economy. Putting money into preventative care, public health initiatives, and easily accessible healthcare strengthens community resilience while also protecting people. A culture that places a high priority on health creates an atmosphere in which people may flourish, be creative, and make significant contributions to the advancement of society. Modern developments in lifestyle awareness, technology, and medical sciences provide never-before-seen chances to improve health. The instruments available for preserving and improving health are varied and constantly changing, ranging from wearable technology that monitors and promotes well-being to tailored treatment. Furthermore, the inclusion of preventative measures shows that proactive health activities are important everywhere, as seen by the incorporation of vaccination programs and public health education. To sum up, the idea of preserving and improving health is a dynamic and complex undertaking that affects society structures and promotes well-being on a worldwide scale. Fostering a resilient and vibrant environment requires an understanding of how physical, mental, and social health are intertwined. Adopting a holistic approach to health becomes not just a personal decision but also a group obligation for the improvement of mankind as we negotiate the complexity of the modern world.

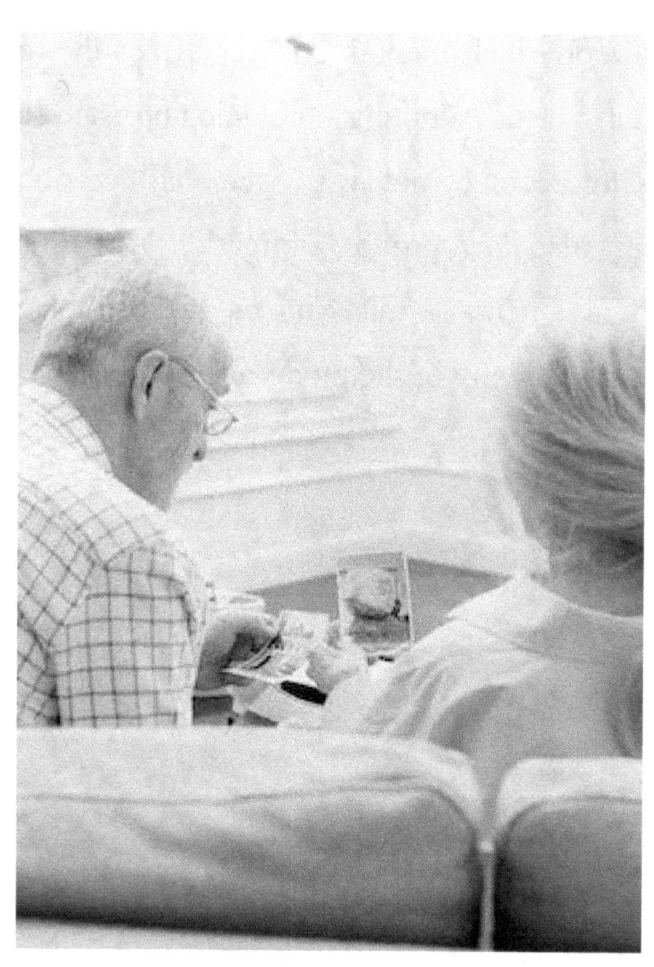

Chapter 1: Understanding Longevity

Definition and significance

When referring to a person's lifespan in the context of human life, longevity mostly refers to an individual's long and healthy lifespan. It encompasses the quality and vibrancy of the years lived, going beyond just survival. Longevity has enormous importance for people since it affects many aspects of personal happiness, social systems, and life in general. Longevity is personally correlated with the chance to have a more rich and satisfying life. It gives people the chance to see and take part in the fabric of their lives as it unfolds, giving them time for introspection, goal-setting, and the development of deep connections. Living a longer life allows one to gain wisdom, a greater awareness of the world and oneself, and a variety of experiences. From the standpoint of health, the quest for long life has sparked breakthroughs in healthcare and the medical sciences. In addition to increasing life expectancy, researchers work to improve the quality of those extra years. Advances in individualized healthcare, preventative medicine, and novel therapies for age-related disorders have resulted from this, which has eventually made the world's population healthier and more resilient. Equally important is the effect that longevity has on society. Longer lifespans challenge conventional ideas about schooling, professional paths, and retirement, changing population patterns. The demands of an aging population force societies to adjust, tackling intergenerational dynamics, social support networks, and healthcare infrastructure, among other things. Additionally, a workforce with a longer lifespan helps support stability and productivity in the economy. Longevity fosters a feeling of continuity and communal memory, connecting generations in the larger human experience. It makes it possible to transmit values, customs, and information from one generation to the next. Humanity's natural drive for advancement, self-improvement, and the never-ending search for a higher standard of living is reflected in the goal of a longer and healthier life. In summary, human longevity is extremely important for a variety of reasons, including personal satisfaction, medical progress, cultural changes, and the transfer of human experience from one generation to the next. In order to shape healthcare practices, individual decisions, and policies that support a robust and vibrant human civilization, it is imperative that we acknowledge and comprehend the complex nature of longevity.

Factors influencing longevity

The amount of time and quality of human existence are shaped by a number of interrelated elements that affect longevity. Comprehending these variables offers valuable perspectives on the intricacies of longevity, which include genetics, lifestyle, medical treatment, and environmental aspects.

1. Genetics: The influence of genetics is crucial in establishing a person's susceptibility to specific illnesses and their average lifespan. Genetic changes, for instance, might affect a person's vulnerability to diseases like diabetes, heart disease, or some forms of cancer. Although genetics establishes the starting point, lifestyle decisions can modify these genetic influences.

2. Lifestyle Choices: Habits, exercise, and diet all have a big influence on lifespan. Consuming a well-rounded and nourishing diet lowers the chance of developing chronic illnesses and improves general health.

Regular exercise has been linked to improved mental, physical, and cardiovascular health. On the other hand, bad behaviors like smoking and binge drinking can reduce life expectancy.

3. Access to Healthcare: Longevity is influenced by the accessibility and availability of healthcare services. Living a longer and healthier life can be attributed to medical breakthroughs, timely treatments, and access to preventative care. Life expectancy may be shortened in areas with poor access to healthcare because of insufficient treatment and preventative measures.

4. Socioeconomic Status: There is a correlation between longevity and

socioeconomic characteristics such as employment, income, and education. Better access to healthcare, healthier lifestyle choices, and less exposure to environmental dangers are frequently linked to higher socioeconomic classes. Contrarily, poverty can shorten life expectancy by limiting access to necessary resources and medical treatment.

5. Environmental Factors: Longevity is influenced by environmental factors, both natural and man-made. Improving access to sanitary facilities, clean water, and air leads to improved health results. Adverse impacts may arise from exposure to pollutants, environmental toxins, or unhealthy living circumstances. Geographical and climatic

variables also affect the prevalence of sickness and general well-being.

6. Social Connections: Longevity has been associated with robust social networks and significant connections. Social interaction and emotional support are factors in mental health that can affect physical health. On the other hand, loneliness and social isolation may be detrimental to one's lifespan and general health.

7. Knowledge and Education: Education provides people with information on illness prevention, healthy lifestyle choices, and healthcare accessibility. Longer life expectancy and better health outcomes are frequently linked to higher education levels.

People who are educated are better able to make decisions regarding their health.

8. Cultural and Lifestyle Practices: Within certain societies, cultural practices and lifestyle standards might have an impact on lifespan. Communities that consume a diet high in fruits, vegetables, and whole grains, for example, may have a lower incidence of some illnesses, which extends their life expectancy.

For the purpose of creating plans to encourage good aging and increase lifespan, it is essential to comprehend the complex interactions between these variables. Living a longer and more satisfying life can be facilitated by adopting a holistic approach that takes into account social, environmental, genetic, and lifestyle factors.

Myths and misconceptions about aging

There are many myths and misconceptions regarding aging in society, which frequently serve to reinforce stereotypes and mold perceptions of senior citizens. The idea that cognitive function will eventually deteriorate with age is one common misconception. Even though age-related cognitive impairments like reduced processing speed are possible, mental stimulation, a healthy lifestyle, and lifelong learning can help older people keep their wits fresh. Another misunderstanding is that elderly individuals are often feeble and incapable of participating in physical pursuits. Actually, regular exercise may improve general well-being, strength, and flexibility, enabling older people to lead active and satisfying lives.

Furthermore, it is false to assume that all seniors lack technical proficiency; rather, many of them welcome and adjust to new technology, defying the myth that they are innately averse to change. Another common misconception is that workers who are older are less flexible and productive than those who are younger. In actuality, senior workers frequently provide invaluable knowledge, sharp problem-solving abilities, and a solid work ethic. Growing older does not always translate into less creativity or productivity. It's a fallacy that growing older means being alone all the time. Many older people maintain strong social ties through family, friends, and community activity, even if their social groups may alter over time.

Regardless of age, it is critical to understand that social involvement is necessary for mental health. Furthermore, it is untrue to assume that elderly people are in stable financial situations. Many people struggle financially, and preconceived notions about wealth can keep disparities alive. Developing successful policies and support systems for older individuals requires an understanding of the variety of financial circumstances that they face. Finally, prospects for lifelong learning are hampered by the myth that elderly individuals are incapable of learning new things. Studies show that people's brains are malleable and that they may keep learning new things throughout their lives. Neglecting the ability to learn as one ages restricts one's ability to advance personally. It is essential to dispel these myths and prejudices in order to promote an age- and inclusion-friendly society. A more realistic portrayal of the talents and experiences of older people, as well as better policies and intergenerational relationships, can result from embracing a comprehensive view of aging.

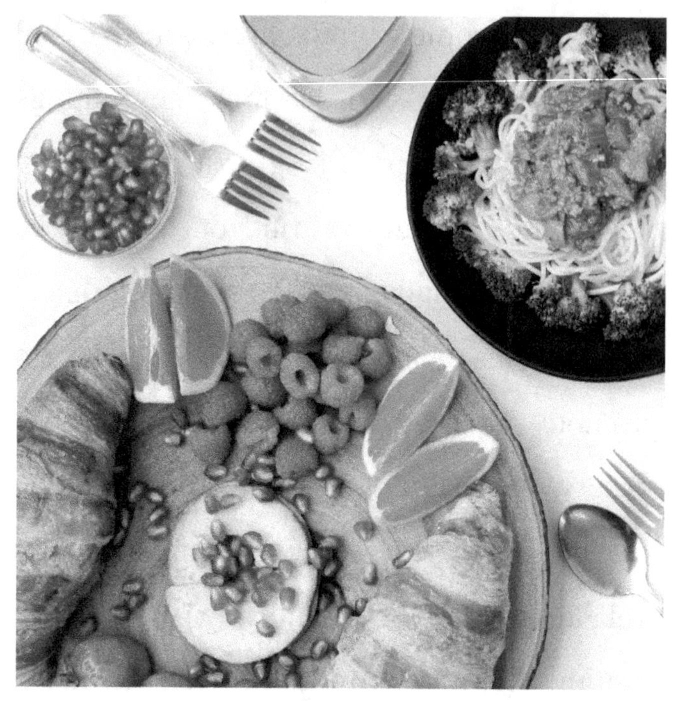

Chapter 2: Foundations of a Healthy Lifestyle

Nutritious diet and its impact on longevity

A healthy diet is essential for extending life since it affects many elements of health and lowers the risk of chronic illnesses. The following are some significant effects of a healthy diet on lifespan, accompanied by examples:

1. Disease Prevention: Essential nutrients and antioxidants that help prevent chronic illnesses are provided by a balanced diet full of fruits, vegetables, whole grains, lean meats, and healthy fats. For instance, a decreased risk of heart disease and several

malignancies has been associated with the Mediterranean diet, which is rich in plant foods, nuts, seafood, and olive oil.

2. Heart Conditions: Eating meals low in cholesterol, salt, saturated fats, and trans fats promotes cardiovascular health. Focusing on fruits, vegetables, lean meats, and low-fat dairy, the Dietary Approaches to Stop Hypertension (DASH) diet has been linked to lowered blood pressure and a lower risk of heart disease.

3. Brain Function: Diets high in nutrients promote mental clarity and may lower the chance of developing neurodegenerative illnesses. Nuts, seeds, and fish are good sources of omega-3 fatty acids, which are known to have neuroprotective effects on

the brain and may lengthen life expectancy by maintaining cognitive function.

4. Weight Control: Longevity depends on eating a balanced diet and maintaining a healthy weight. Numerous health problems, such as diabetes and cardiovascular disorders, are associated with obesity. Including foods high in fiber, such as legumes and whole grains, can aid in boosting satiety and weight control.

5. Immune System Support: Foods abundant in nutrients, especially vitamins and minerals, help maintain a strong immune system. The body fights infections and maintains general health when it gets enough zinc from nuts and seeds and vitamin C from fruits like citrus and berries.

6. Cellular Health: Fruits and vegetables include antioxidants that help fight oxidative stress, which can cause illness and aging. Rich in antioxidants, berries, leafy greens, and vibrant veggies can help shield cells from harm.

7. Health of the Gut: A healthy gut microbiome is encouraged by a diet high in fiber from fruits, vegetables, and whole grains. Overall health is enhanced by a healthy microbiome, which is associated with better nutrition absorption, better digestion, and a lower risk of inflammatory diseases.

8. Skull Health: Maintaining bone health requires consuming enough calcium and vitamin D, which are frequently present in dairy products and meals that have been

fortified. As one ages, this becomes increasingly important in preventing fractures and osteoporosis.

In conclusion, eating a varied diet rich in nutrient-dense foods has a good effect on general health, lowers the risk of chronic illnesses, and lengthens life. Dietary patterns that promote longevity, such as the DASH and Mediterranean diets, demonstrate how important it is to follow certain dietary guidelines to maintain good health and wellbeing over the long term.

Importance of regular physical activity

Frequent physical activity has a positive impact on many elements of both physical and mental health, which is essential for prolonging a lifespan. The following are some of the main arguments for why regular exercise is essential for living a longer and healthier life, along with some instances of these advantages:

1. Health of the Heart: Frequent exercise lowers the risk of cardiovascular disorders by strengthening the heart and enhancing blood circulation. Exercises that improve cardiovascular fitness, such as cycling, running, and brisk walking, reduce the risk of heart attacks and strokes.

2. Weight Control: Maintaining a healthy weight requires physical activity. Exercises that burn calories and maintain a healthy body weight, such as swimming, strength

training, or jogging, lower the risk of obesity-related diseases like type 2 diabetes.

3. Healthy Joints and Bone Density: Walking, hiking, and weightlifting are examples of weight-bearing workouts that help to preserve joint health and bone density. This is crucial for maintaining general mobility as people age and preventing osteoporosis.

4. Healthy Metabolism: By increasing insulin sensitivity and regulating blood sugar better, exercise lowers the risk of type 2 diabetes. Regular aerobic exercise and high-intensity interval training (HIIT) are two examples of activities that effectively improve metabolic health.

5. Intellectual Function: Engaging in regular physical activity helps maintain brain function and lowers the chance of age-related cognitive deterioration. Improved cognitive function is a result of physical and mental involvement in activities such as dance.

6. Psychological Health: One effective strategy for lowering stress and enhancing mental health is exercise. In addition to enhancing mental health and physical fitness, practices like yoga and mindfulness-based exercises also improve overall life happiness.

7. Support for Immune Systems: The immune system is strengthened by moderate exercise, such as brisk walking or

moderate-intensity cycling. Frequent exercise strengthens the immune system and aids in the body's defense against illnesses.

8. Enhanced Rest: Improved sleep quality is associated with physical exercise. Participating in activities such as mild yoga or moderate aerobic workouts encourages relaxation and helps to enhance sleep patterns.

9. "Solidarity by Social Involvement Social connection is a key component of many physical activities, which promotes a sense of community. Participating in group activities such as hiking groups, team sports, or fitness courses offers chances for social interaction and can lead to a longer and more satisfying life.

10. Flexibility and Balance: Exercises that emphasize balance and flexibility, like tai chi or yoga, are crucial for avoiding falls and preserving mobility as one ages, supporting an active and independent lifestyle.

To sum up, consistent physical exercise enhances cardiovascular health, helps control weight, maintains bone density, improves mental and emotional health, boosts the immune system, and much more. Including a variety of fitness activities in one's routine guarantees a comprehensive approach to health, which promotes a longer and healthier life.

Mental well-being and its connection to longevity

Longevity and mental health are closely related because psychological health has a big impact on physical health and, in turn, life expectancy. Many studies indicate that people who have strong mental health also often live longer, and there are a number of factors that may be involved in this association.

First, habits that affect lifespan are influenced by mental health. For example, those who have healthy lifestyles—such as frequent exercise, a balanced diet, and adequate sleep—are more likely to be in excellent mental health. These actions enhance general physical health, lower the chance of developing chronic diseases, and eventually lengthen life expectancy. On the other hand, people who are dealing with mental health concerns may develop bad behaviors, which makes them more susceptible to other health conditions.

Second, there is a significant effect of stress on lifespan. Prolonged stress can hasten aging by causing physiological reactions that are frequently associated with poor mental health. Increased amounts of stress hormones such as cortisol can cause cardiovascular problems, inflammation, and weakened immune systems, all of which have an impact on life expectancy. Conversely, strong mental health can help to effectively manage stress and counteract these negative consequences, eventually leading to improved health results.

Social ties are also very important. People who possess robust social support networks, which are an essential element of mental health, typically exhibit reduced stress levels and heightened resilience. These elements support a longer life and better physical health. For instance, compared to seniors who lead socially isolated lifestyles, those who keep active social lives may benefit from improved cognitive function and a lower risk of chronic illnesses.

Moreover, a healthy mental state has a direct impact on the body's capacity to heal from disease and age. Immune system performance and cellular healing mechanisms have been related to positive psychological emotions like hope and purpose. On the other hand, disorders that can shorten life expectancy have been linked to compromised immune responses and conditions such as depression.

In summary, there are a variety of relationships between lifespan and mental health. Good mental health encourages good habits, lessens the negative effects of stress, strengthens social bonds, and improves the body's capacity to withstand aging and disease. So, it is essential to comprehend and take care of mental health in order to prolong a healthy and meaningful life, as well as to enhance life quality.

Chapter 3: Simple Habits for Longevity

Daily routines for health maintenance

Incorporating daily routines that focus on one's physical, mental, and emotional well-being is essential to maintaining a healthy lifestyle. This thorough guide will assist you in creating a balanced routine for maintaining your health, complete with examples.

1. Morning Hydration: To rehydrate and speed up metabolism, have a glass of water as soon as you wake up. - As an illustration,

drink warm water with a lemon slice for more antioxidants.

2.   Nutrient-Rich   Breakfast: Eat   a well-balanced breakfast that includes fiber, protein, and good fats. For instance, Greek yogurt is topped with chia seeds and berries.

3. Regular Exercise: Include a minimum of thirty minutes of physical exercise, such as weight training, yoga, or running. For instance, a jog in the morning or a workout at home.

4. Mindful Meditation: Set aside time for mindfulness meditation to improve mental clarity and lower stress. For instance, use concentrated breathing techniques or guided meditation.

5. Healthy Snacking: Select nutrient-dense snacks in between meals, such as veggies, fruits, or almonds. Slices of apple with almond butter, for instance.

6. Hydration Throughout the Day: To keep hydrated, try to have at least 8 glasses of water throughout the day. For diversity, try infused water or herbal teas.

7. "Well-Rounded Lunch Choose a lunch that is well-rounded by including whole grains, lean meats, and vibrant veggies. For instance, stir-fried vegetables, quinoa, and grilled chicken.

8. Stretch pauses: Take quick pauses from your job to stretch and prevent sitting for

extended periods of time. For instance, standing desk exercises or stretches for the neck and shoulders.

9. Healthy Afternoon Snack: Pick foods that keep you full for a long time, such as a handful of mixed nuts. For instance, hummus and carrot sticks.

10. Evening Relaxation: Take a warm bath or read a book to unwind in the evening. For instance, a good book and herbal tea.

11. Nutrient-Packed Dinner: Choose a filling, light supper that includes lots of vegetables and lean meats. For instance, baked salmon is served with quinoa and steamed broccoli.

12. Screen Time Limits: Establish guidelines for screen time before bed in order to enhance the quality of your sleep. As an illustration, turn off all electronics an hour before bed.

13. Adequate Sleep: For general wellbeing, aim for 7-9 hours of good sleep per night. For instance, create a regular bedtime schedule.

14. Thankfulness Practice: Write in a thankfulness notebook about the good things that happened during the day. For instance, list three things for which you are thankful.

15. Social Connections: Develop deep connections to promote emotional health.

Example: Consistent phone conversations or get-togethers with loved ones.

You may create a long-term, well-rounded approach to health maintenance by implementing these behaviors into your everyday routine.

Incorporating mindfulness practices

By enhancing general wellbeing, including thoughtful behaviors in your lifestyle can have a positive effect on your lifespan.

Keeping a nutritious and well-balanced diet is essential. Accept entire meals that are high in minerals, vitamins, and antioxidants. Give fruits, vegetables, lean meats, and whole grains a priority while reducing your intake of processed foods and added sugar.

Another important component is regular physical activity. Take part in something you love doing, like yoga, weight training, or brisk walking. Exercise is essential for a happy and longer life since it not only promotes physical health but also enhances mood and cognitive performance.

Efficient sleep is essential for a long life. Make sure your bedroom is restful, stick to a regular sleep schedule, and have a calming nighttime ritual. Adequate sleep is beneficial for the immune system, brain health, and general well-being.

Stress reduction methods and mindfulness are crucial. Include yoga, deep breathing techniques, or meditation in your everyday practice. Learning how to reduce and manage stress is essential for long-term health since chronic stress can have detrimental effects on one's health.

Developing social ties is an additional important component. Develop deep and meaningful bonds with your loved ones. Emotional well-being is enhanced by social support, which also has a favorable impact on physical and mental health.

Longevity depends on ongoing education and mental challenges. Take up mentally taxing hobbies like reading, solving puzzles, or picking up a new skill. As you age, maintaining cognitive function may be achieved by keeping your brain engaged.

Preventive care and routine health examinations are essential. Keep an eye on your health, take quick action to treat any concerns, and take preventative steps to ward off possible problems.

Although it's sometimes forgotten, staying hydrated is essential to general health. Make sure you consume enough water each day to sustain your body's processes and keep your health at its best.

In conclusion, improving lifespan necessitates a comprehensive strategy. Eat healthily, move your body frequently, get enough sleep, handle stress in a thoughtful manner, build relationships with others, keep your mind occupied, take proactive care of your health, and drink enough water. Together, these mindful practices support a longer, healthier, and happier life with the potential for greater longevity.

Quality sleep and its role in longevity

Longevity is largely dependent on getting enough sleep, which affects both physical and mental health in different ways. A robust immune system is associated with enough restorative sleep, which lowers the likelihood of diseases that might compromise general health.

Additionally, it supports efficient memory consolidation, emotional control, and cognitive function—all critical components of preserving a good standard of living as one ages. Furthermore, sleep has a profound effect on hormone balance and weight management, and it is closely linked to metabolic health.

Chronic sleep deprivation has been linked to a higher chance of developing illnesses, including diabetes, obesity, and cardiovascular disorders, all of which can shorten one's life expectancy. Furthermore, the body regenerates and repairs itself when in deep sleep, which helps to maintain organs and tissues.

The ability to restore is essential for long-term health. Stress hormone regulation is aided by sleep, and prolonged stress has been connected to a number of health problems. In conclusion, getting enough sleep is essential for living a long life, as it affects the immune system, mental clarity, metabolic balance, and general wellbeing. Making enough time for quality, restful sleep is essential to living a long and healthy life.

Chapter 4: Avoiding Detrimental Practices

Identifying and eliminating harmful habits

A number of bad behaviors can seriously shorten life expectancy and negatively affect general health. Promoting a longer and healthier life depends on recognizing and breaking these patterns.

1. Tobacco use: Numerous ailments, such as lung cancer, cardiovascular problems, and respiratory disorders, are significantly

influenced by smoking. One of the most significant measures for increasing longevity is giving up smoking.

2. Overindulgence in Alcohol: Long-term alcohol misuse can cause cardiovascular problems, liver damage, and an increased risk of developing certain malignancies. The key to enhancing longevity in alcohol consumption is moderation or removal.

3. Unhealthy Diet: Obesity, diabetes, and heart disease are caused by eating a diet heavy in processed foods, saturated fats, and refined sugars. Choosing a diet rich in fruits, vegetables, whole grains, and other nutrients, along with balance, promotes longevity and good health.

4. A Sedentary Way of Life: A lack of exercise has been connected to a number of health problems, such as heart disease, obesity, and weakening of the muscles and bones. Maintaining a healthy weight, cardiovascular health, and general life span all depend on regular exercise.

5. Not Getting Enough Sleep: Lack of sleep for an extended period of time can harm the immune system, impair cognition, and raise the chance of developing chronic illnesses. Getting enough good sleep is essential for long-term health and well-being.

6. Persistent Stress: Extended periods of stress have been linked to a number of health concerns, such as immune system deficiencies, heart difficulties, and mental

health disorders. Longevity depends on implementing stress-reduction strategies like mindfulness and relaxation training.

7. Poor Portion Control and Overeating: Overindulging in calories can exacerbate obesity and its associated health problems. Maintaining a healthy weight and promoting longevity can be achieved through mindful eating and portion management practices.

8. Ignoring Mental Health: Ignoring mental health can have an adverse effect on general health. Anxiety, sadness, and chronic stress are associated with a number of physical health problems. A longer and better life depends on getting mental health help when required.

9. Dangerous Sunlight Exposure: Without protection, prolonged sun exposure can cause skin damage and raise the chance of developing skin cancer. The lifespan and health of your skin depend on wearing protective clothes and sunscreen.

10. Ignoring Routine Medical Exams: Regular health checkups should not be neglected, as this might lead to hidden health problems. Better long-term health can be promoted by routine screenings and check-ups, which can assist in identifying and addressing possible issues early.

It takes awareness, dedication, and lifestyle adjustments to break these bad behaviors. You may live a longer and healthier life by embracing healthy practices and asking for help when you need it.

Creating a sustainable health plan

A long-term, sustainable health plan must include a balanced approach to mental health, physical exercise, diet, and preventative care.

Frequent exercise promotes general health and lowers the risk of chronic illnesses, including strength and cardiovascular training.

Essential nutrients and antioxidants may be obtained via a plant-based diet high in fruits, vegetables, and whole grains. For the body to operate at its best, drinking alcohol in moderation and staying well hydrated are important.

Emotional resilience is promoted when mental health is prioritized via stress reduction, restful sleep, and mindfulness exercises. Frequent tests and check-ups for health problems can identify any problems early.

Important preventative actions include abstaining from tobacco use and limiting exposure to environmental contaminants.

Emotional well-being is improved by strong support networks and social ties. A fulfilled life is the result of pursuing interests and maintaining a work-life balance. Cognitive health is supported by ongoing learning and mental stimulation, whether via educational opportunities or interesting hobbies.

In the end, living a steady, holistic lifestyle is what leads to longevity. This long-term strategy emphasizes prevention, comprehensive self-care, and preserving a happy, encouraging atmosphere.

Chapter 5: Embracing Aging with Grace

Changing perspectives on aging

Changing older people's perceptions of aging entails encouraging an optimistic and self-empowering view of the aging process.

First and foremost, it's critical to support a mentality change that embraces life's inevitable course. This entails showcasing the wisdom and worth that come with age, as well as the special insights and life experience that older people offer to their communities.

Achieving a shift in self-perception requires encouraging active and healthy aging. Maintaining vitality may be achieved by promoting frequent physical exercise that is tailored to each person's skills and interests.

Providing chances for lifelong learning and skill enhancement strengthens a feeling of achievement and purpose, refuting the idea that growing older means a deterioration in one's skills. In order to promote a sense of belonging and fight feelings of isolation, it is important to establish solid social relationships.

Programs in the community that encourage social interaction and networks of support might help foster a positive attitude about aging. In addition to preserving cultural and historical information, encouraging older people to share their experiences and tales helps to perpetuate the notion that aging is a dynamic and ever-evolving aspect of life.

Moreover, giving people opportunities to engage in society and make significant contributions helps dispel the myth that aging is a time of dependency or idleness. Participating in community activities, volunteering, and serving as a mentor demonstrate the continued significance and influence of senior citizens. It is imperative that ageism in healthcare be addressed.

Instead of concentrating just on treating illnesses, healthcare providers should use a holistic approach that emphasizes preserving functional independence and general well-being. This method serves to promote the notion that aging is a varied and natural process that may be assisted by providing individualized care.

In conclusion, encouraging a positive outlook, supporting active and healthy lives, cultivating social connections, offering chances for significant contributions, and tackling ageism in healthcare are all important aspects of helping the elderly change their perceptions of aging. Societies may encourage a more happy and satisfying experience for folks in their later years by embracing the natural characteristics of aging and emphasizing the continuous significance of older individuals.

Balancing natural methods with medical interventions

The aim of aging gracefully and extending life spans through a holistic strategy that takes into account both lifestyle choices and improvements in healthcare involves striking a balance between natural techniques and medicinal treatments. Through the combination of these tactics, people can maximize their well-being. Natural approaches include a variety of lifestyle decisions, such as stress reduction, a balanced diet, frequent exercise, and enough sleep.

An antioxidant-, vitamin-, and mineral-rich, well-balanced diet can promote cellular health and lessen the effects of oxidative stress, a major cause of aging. Frequent exercise has been connected to enhanced cardiovascular health, increased muscular strength, and enhanced cognitive performance, all of which extend life expectancy.

Stress reduction techniques like mindfulness and meditation have a positive effect on mental health and may even slow down the aging process. A longer, healthier life may be attained by getting enough sleep, which is essential for immune system support and cellular renewal.

Interventions, including regenerative treatments, customized medicine, and preventative screenings, are important in the medical field. Personalized medicine maximizes efficacy and reduces negative effects by customizing care based on a patient's genetic composition. With the goal of mending and revitalizing tissues, regenerative therapies—which include stem cell treatments—may be able to halt the aging process and lessen the effects of age-related illnesses.

Early diagnosis and action are made possible by preventive screenings, which include routine physical examinations and screens for diseases including cancer and cardiovascular disease. This proactive strategy can have a major effect on results and lengthen lifespans.

Combining a plant-based diet high in anti-inflammatory foods with regular cardiovascular activity is an example of this integrated strategy in action. While medical measures such as cholesterol-lowering drugs or enhanced cardiovascular tests might further increase heart health, this natural strategy enhances overall health.

In a similar vein, social interaction and cognitive workouts are organic ways to promote brain health. This integrated approach tackles the complex nature of aging in combination with medical interventions such as neuroprotective medicines or pharmaceuticals that enhance cognitive function. Ultimately, the secret to a holistic approach to aging and lifespan is the synergy between medical interventions and natural techniques. With the help of this integrated approach, people may take advantage of the advantages of both modern medical breakthroughs and lifestyle choices, forging a sustainable and balanced route to a longer, healthier life.

Inspirational anecdotes of individuals who achieved longevity

1. Miselu Harada (first name): Miselu, who is 116 years old, credits her passion for painting, a plant-based diet, and regular

walks for her life. She thought that her long, happy life was a result of her pursuit of her artistic interests and being active.

2. Jiroemon Kimura, who lived to 116 years old, is known as the oldest man in history. His basic diet, fewer amounts, and keeping socially engaged in his community all contributed to his longevity, which he attributed to these factors.

3. The following is Emma Morano: Emma Morano, who lived to be 117 years old, said that her diet of raw eggs and her optimistic attitude toward life were her secrets. Her ability to bounce back from personal setbacks demonstrated the value of having a strong spirit in living a long life.

4. The author, Shigeaki Hinohara Hinohara, a 105-year-old Japanese doctor, stressed the need for a balanced diet, regular exercise, and finding fulfillment in one's career. His extraordinary lifespan was facilitated by his dedication to inquiry and continual study.

5. Rose-colored Brown: Violet Brown, who lived to be 117 years old, attributed her long life to perseverance, faith, and a diet high in fruits and vegetables that were grown nearby. Those around her were motivated by her dedication to upholding a robust work ethic and a healthy lifestyle.

6. Luigi Cornaro, the sixth: Luigi Cornaro was a Venetian nobleman of the fifteenth century who lived to reach an astonishing ninety-eight years old. He emphasized a

balanced and disciplined lifestyle and supported eating and drinking in moderation.

7. Christopher Coke: Nicholas Coke, who lived to be 108 years old, credited his long life to keeping a happy attitude, remaining active in society, and appreciating the small things in life, such as gardening and spending time with loved ones.

8. Mushatt Jones, Susannah: Susannah Mushatt Jones, who was 116 years old, attributed her long and happy life to having a profound sense of humor, a close family relationship, and a daily dosage of bacon.

9. Lumbreras, Leandra Becerra: Leandra, who claimed to be 127 years old, attributed

her long life to a diet free of processed foods and alcohol, regular exercise, and a strong sense of community and faith that she upheld throughout her years.

10. LaPallo Bernardo: Bernando LaPallo, who lived to reach 114 years old, credited his long life to daily exercise, a diet high in fresh fruits and vegetables, and an optimistic outlook. In order to live a full and vibrant life, he underlined the significance of taking care of the body and mind.

Conclusion, encouragement and call to action

In the quest for longevity, the narratives of those who have gone beyond traditional age norms provide motivation. These stories highlight the variety of approaches one may take to live a longer, better life, from centenarians who like taking daily walks to nonagenarians who appreciate the ease of a balanced diet. Upon contemplating the insights imparted by those who have achieved extraordinary longevity, it is apparent that the secrets of long life transcend the number of years and instead involve holistic health, intentional lifestyles, and an optimistic outlook.

Longevityty is defined not only by the number of years lived but also by the standard of living in those years. Being long-lived is not only a biological achievement; it is also a reflection of the decisions we make on a daily basis, the connections we form, and the fortitude with which we confront life's obstacles.

The centenarians and supercentenarians that these stories highlight did not find the fountain of youth; instead, they deliberately pursued lives that supported their mental, emotional, and physical health. A consistent theme across these tales is the significance placed on eating a well-rounded and nourishing diet.

Food is central to the story of longevity, from Miselu Harada's plant-based diet to Nicholas Coke's moderation. The basis for a strong immune system and a healthy body is consuming full, nutrient-rich meals while avoiding overindulgence. The takeaway is unambiguous: our dietary choices have a big influence on the energy we derive from life.

The need to maintain an active lifestyle throughout your life is equally vital. Engaging in physical exercise, such as walking, cycling, or meaningful employment, is a key component of longevity. The transforming value of being physically active is attested to by Shigeaki Hinohara's dedication to movement and Jiroemon Kimura's modest workout regimen. Frequent exercise strengthens the connection between the mind and body by promoting mental clarity, emotional stability, and cardiovascular health.

The stories emphasize the value of having a good outlook and a sense of purpose in life, even outside of the physical world. Luigi Cornaro's moderation philosophy, Emma Morano's constant optimism, and Bernando LaPallo's emphasis on a positive attitude highlight the transforming power of developing a resilient mindset. A sense of purpose that transcends age may be achieved by pursuing lifelong learning, participating in enjoyable activities, and building strong social relationships. As we take in the wisdom of these extraordinary people, a call to action becomes apparent.

The route to longevity is not an illusive destination that only a few choose; rather, it is a call to action for all of us to make deliberate decisions in our day-to-day existence. The call to action is a request to set out on a path of longevity, equipped with the understanding that gradual, minor adjustments may have a significant impact.

Start by evaluating the foods you eat, the amount of exercise you get, and the mentality you cultivate as part of your lifestyle choices. Adopt a healthy, well-balanced diet that includes a range of whole foods that will benefit your body. Find things to do that make you happy and uplift your spirits, and incorporate regular physical exercise into your schedule. Develop an optimistic outlook, understanding the importance of optimism in adjusting to the ups and downs of life. It is never too early or too late to begin creating a plan for your path toward longevity.

The decisions you make now will have an impact on your health and well-being in the future. Being long-lived is a journey that never ends, requiring self-care and enjoyment of the energy that comes with a life well-lived. When you start along the path to longevity, think about the kind of legacy you want to leave behind—one that isn't only measured in years but also in the depth of connections, the breadth of experiences, and the happiness that comes from living a life that has meaning. Allow the experiences of those who have gone before you to influence and direct your decisions. May resilience, well-being, and purpose weave together to create a timeless masterpiece in the fabric of your life.

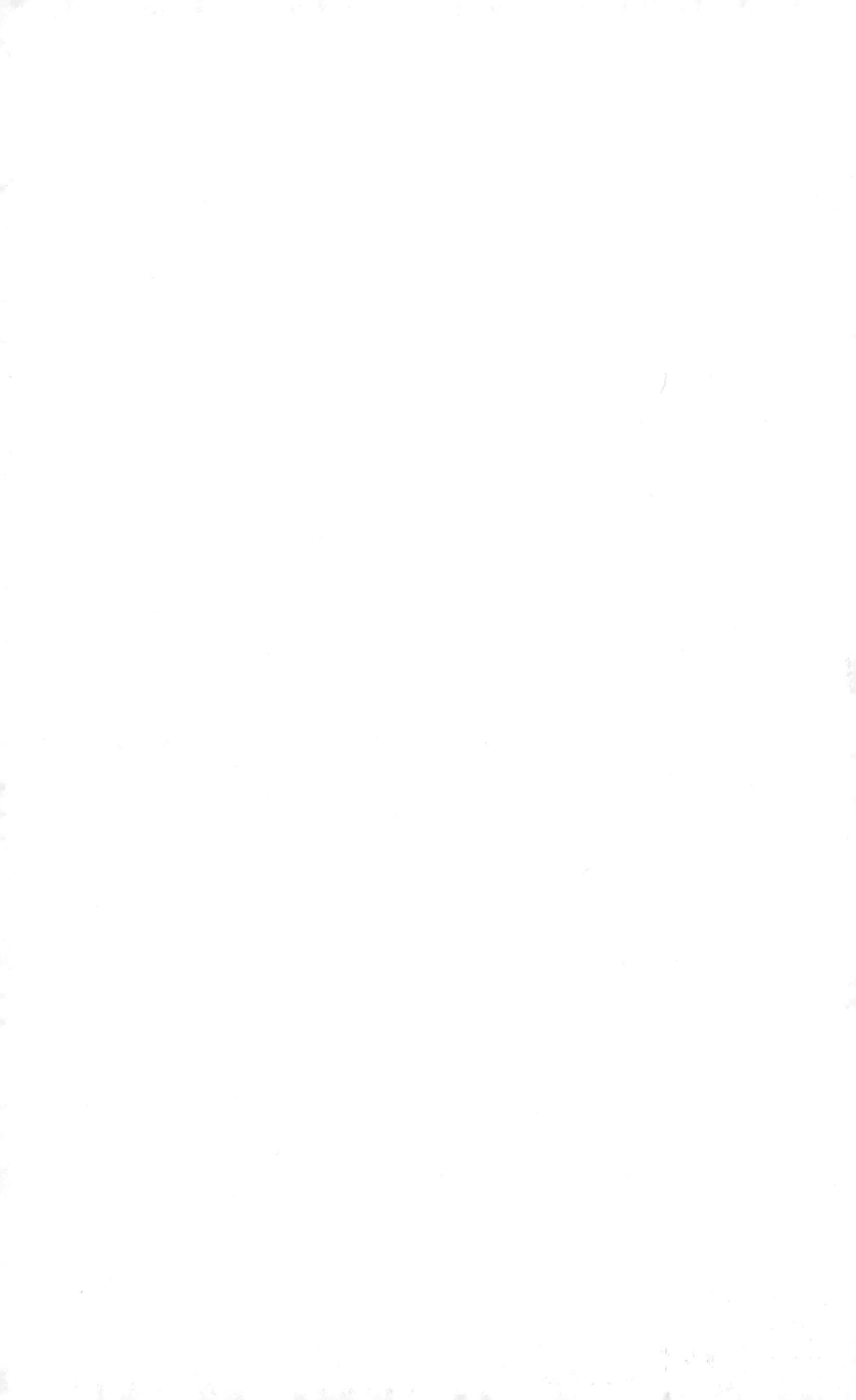